Proven Alternative Ways to Heal Common Chronic Digestive Problems:

What Your Doctor Doesn't Know Can Keep You From Healing

By Helen Chin Lui,

Certified Reflexologist, Certified Energy Medicine & Reiki Practitioner

Proven Alternative Ways to Heal Common Chronic Digestive Problems: What Your Doctor Doesn't Know Can Keep You From Healing
by Helen Chin Lui, Copyright © February, 2013
Published by Healing Place Medfield

First Edition. Printed and bound in the United States of America.

ISBN-13: 978-0615769349
ISBN-10: 0615769349 9 8 7 6 5 4 3 2

Chin Lui, Helen
Proven Alternative Ways to Heal Common Chronic Digestive Problems: What Your Doctor Doesn't Know Can Keep You From Healing

Digestive Health
Proven Alternative Ways to Heal Common Chronic Digestive Problems: What Your Doctor Doesn't Know Can Keep You From Healing
by Helen Chin Lui

IBS
Proven Alternative Ways to Heal Common Chronic Digestive Problems: What Your Doctor Doesn't Know Can Keep You From Healing
by Helen Chin Lui

Holistic Digestive Health
Proven Alternative Ways to Heal Common Chronic Digestive Problems: What Your Doctor Doesn't Know Can Keep You From Healing
by Helen Chin Lui

For all my Clients with Digestive Health Issues

Proven Alternative Ways to Heal Common Chronic Digestive Problems:

What Your Doctor Doesn't Know Can Keep You From Healing

By Helen Chin Lui,
Certified Reflexologist, Certified Energy Medicine & Reiki Practitioner

Thank you for purchasing this booklet on Digestive Health. My name is Helen Chin Lui. I am the owner and founder of the Healing Place in Medfield, Massachusetts. I am a certified Reflexologist, Energy Medicine, and Reiki practitioner, performing therapeutic energy healing since 2006. My specialty is helping clients find relief from chronic digestive disorders.

Digestive disorder statistics in 2004 [1]

- Over $12 billion is spent on various digestive medications annually
- There were more than 104 million people admitted to hospitals for digestive disorders
- White females between the ages 15-65+ are affected by digestive disorder more frequently..
- 236,164 deaths were documented as due to digestive disorder diseases

What will this booklet cover?

The information in this booklet as compiled over a six year period as a Reflexologist, Energy Medicine and Reiki practitioner, from my past and current clients' digestive disorder experiences. I have seen men, women, teens, children and infants with various digestive disorders consisting mostly of constipation, acid reflux, indigestion and/or irritable bowel syndrome (IBS) issues.

These clients:

- Have sought traditional medicine solutions which have not completely helped
- Have exhausted all pharmaceutical means and still have digestive discomfort
- Want to proactively take charge of their own health

I will be discussing common digestive disorder cases that I see at my office on a weekly basis, and how reflexology and energy medicine helps. I will share techniques that you can use safely on your own, although the fastest, most accurate results will happen by working with me directly, either in person, or virtually by Skype. The tips I will be sharing are for informational purposes only, and should not be considered medical advice. Please consult with your healthcare provider before starting any new health regimen.

Table of Contents

Indigestion

Indigestion is the most common digestive system disorder and can be described as pain or discomfort in the upper abdomen. Also known as dyspepsia, acid reflux, or GERD [(2)], indigestion affects about 15% of the population in western countries.

Indigestion is not a disease. Indigestion is a group of symptoms which often include bloating, nausea and burping. It is usually caused by stomach acid coming into contact with the mucosa of the digestive system - the sensitive protective lining. Stomach acids break down the mucosa, causing irritation and inflammation that trigger indigestion symptoms.

What Causes Indigestion?

Indigestion is usually related to lifestyle and what we eat and drink and may be accompanied by other symptoms, such as fullness in the stomach or belching. Sometimes, indigestion can be caused by other factors, such as an infection or taking certain medications. Common causes include:

- Eating too much and/or too fast
- Eating too much chocolate, fatty, and/or spicy foods
- Drinking too much caffeine, alcohol, and/or carbonated drinks
- Gallstones
- Being overweight
- Medication
- Insufficient sleep

Remedy Options

Diet and lifestyle changes - If symptoms are mild and your indigestion is not occurring often, some lifestyle changes will probably ease symptoms. Try consuming less fatty foods, avoiding spicy foods, eliminating caffeine, alcohol, and chocolates and consistently getting a good night's sleep of at least seven hours.

Holistic remedy - A combined ear, hand and foot reflexology therapy is excellent for finding relief for indigestion. Average results are achieved within 3-4 sessions with a professional Reflexologist, followed by a monthly maintenance reflexology program once indigestion is diminished.

Heartburn

Despite the name, heartburn has nothing to do with the heart. It is a digestive problem that occurs when stomach acid comes into contact with the lining of the esophagus and the acid content of the stomach passes backwards up into the food pipe, known also as the gullet or esophagus. This irritation is known as acid reflux. Most people have experienced stomach acid reflux at some point in their lives, either as heartburn or acid regurgitation. Heartburn is annoying and may have a detrimental effect on a person's wellbeing. Sometimes the tendency for heartburn may develop into a mucous membrane inflammation in the food pipe, known as esophagitis. In the worst cases, esophagitis can become complicated with ulcers, which, in rare cases, may bleed or cause chronic anemia. Occasionally, scars from reflux esophagitis cause a tightening or narrowing (stricture) in the food pipe making swallowing difficult. If this should occur, it is a serious condition which requires immediate attention.

What Causes Heartburn?

When the lower esophageal sphincter (LES) - the valve that keeps stomach acid in the stomach - is weakened or relaxed, it does not do its job properly. This is the most common symptom of gastro esophageal reflux disease (GERD). Things that can weaken or relax the LES include:

- Eating certain foods (chocolate, fried and fatty foods, peppermint, coffee, alcohol, and sugars).
- Eating large meals.
- Eating shortly before bedtime.
- Pressure on the stomach, including frequent bending over, tight clothes, lifting, and obesity.
- Some medications.

Heartburn once a month is considered mild and about 20% of all adults do experience monthly symptoms. Weekly symptoms of heartburn are considered moderate and only when your heartburn occurs daily is it considered to be severe.

Remedy Options

You can manage uncomfortable episodes with a change of diet to reduce acidic foods, and/or over-the-counter medications, and/or weight loss. Only 5-15% of severe heartburn sufferers will find partial or temporary relief with these remedies.

Holistic remedy - A combined ear, hand and foot reflexology therapy has helped 100% of my clients find relief from heartburn in a relatively short time. Average results are achieved within 3-4 sessions with a professional Reflexologist followed by a monthly maintenance reflexology program once indigestion is diminished.

Client Observation *– Sam, age 67, has been having regular reflexology sessions since 2006. He has chronic heartburn due to poor eating habits which he prefers to continue. He loves hamburgers and french fries and eats this combination at least two to three times a week. Sam takes antacids to lessen symptoms after they appear. To prevent heartburn, though, Sam watches his diet and comes for bimonthly reflexology sessions. He values his sessions because they greatly lessen the occurrence of heartburn especially when he is off track with his eating.*

Irritable Bowel Syndrome (IBS)

IBS affects 1 in 5 adults in the United States, making it one of the most common ailments diagnosed by doctors. IBS symptoms range from bloating, gas, diarrhea or constipation to the more life-threatening colorectal cancer. They encompass disorders of the gastrointestinal tract, as well as the liver, gallbladder, and pancreas.

IBS is a common digestive system disorder, which simply means 'inflammation of the colon'. While most people experience digestive troubles once in a while, what sets IBS - also known as "spastic colon"- apart is belly pain and diarrhea or constipation that comes back again and again. IBS involves abnormal gut contractions that tend to be chronic, characterized by abdominal pain, bloating, mucous in stools, and irregular bowel habits with alternating diarrhea and constipation symptoms.

What Causes IBS?

The medical field does not know what causes IBS. It is believed that the signals between the brain and intestines are somehow disrupted. This miscommunication may cause abnormal intestinal muscle contractions.

Anyone can develop IBS, but the condition is twice as common in women as in men. It is also more likely to affect people who have a family history of IBS.

Remedy Options

The first step toward managing IBS is to identify what aggravates your symptoms. Besides stress, common triggers include: eating a meal, hormonal changes, and certain medications. It is important to note that no specific foods have been universally linked to IBS symptoms.

Keeping a food diary may help you pinpoint which foods are problems for you. You may find it helpful to avoid caffeine, alcohol, and fatty foods. Getting more fiber or water may also improve symptoms. It is suggested to introduce probiotics or prebiotics and omega oils into your diet. Probiotics or prebiotics are specific types of bacteria that live in the human gut. They are known as friendly bacteria that have been found to relieve lactose intolerance, prevent vaginal and bladder infections and allergies, and also reduce the growth of harmful organisms in the digestive tract. Omega oils help to lubricate and keep food moving smoothly and efficiently through the intestines, thereby encouraging regular, healthy bowel movements. Omega oils provide nourishment to the intestinal lining cells and help to strengthen the intestinal lining and prevent the passage of harmful toxins into the bloodstream. Other treatment options can include medication and lifestyle changes such as diet, exercise, and stress management to control symptoms.

Holistic remedy - A combined Energy Medicine and ear, hand and foot reflexology therapy has helped 90% of my clients to find relief from IBS. Results normally take place within eight sessions with a professional Reflexologist. A monthly reflexology program is suggested once gastrointestinal balance is achieved.

Client Observation – Joan, age 35, has been coming for regular, monthly reflexology sessions since 2008 to help calm her IBS symptoms. Joan is a teacher in a classroom of children under the age of 5. The job of balancing teaching, talking to parents and working with administrators can be extremely taxing to her patience. Upon coming to the Healing Place we determined Joan holds most of her stress in her lower abdominal region. Before reflexology Joan would have monthly IBS flare-ups, after three months of regular reflexology she has reduced that number to two or three IBS flare-ups a year. Joan is pleased with the results of her regular reflexology sessions.

Constipation

Statistics:

- More than 4 million Americans (12-19%) suffer from chronic constipation in the USA (including children, adults and elderly).
- 2.5 million annual doctor's visits are for constipation.
- More than $700 million is spent on over-the-counter laxative products annually.

In a healthy person, the bowels should move at least once a day and Naturopaths suggest we should have a bowel movement after each meal. When we are constipated, the water in the feces is re-absorbed by the body causing the stools to harden in the colon. Eventually, the colon loses its muscle tone and the condition becomes chronic. Symptoms associated with constipation include infrequent bowel movements, hard stools, straining when passing a movement, cramps, abdominal bloating, flatulence, and a desire to defecate but an inability to pass stools.

Remedy Options

Fiber and water should be included in your diet to help promote bowel movements and prevent constipation. There are two main types of fiber, soluble and insoluble. Soluble fiber dissolves in water, insoluble fiber does not. Fiber cannot be digested. Soluble fiber transforms as it passes through the digestive tract, where it is fermented by bacteria. Soluble fiber absorbs water, and becomes gelatinous as it does so. Insoluble fiber passes through the gut without changing its form. In doing so, the fiber sweeps through the intestines acting like a broom to keep food moving along and prevent it from sticking to the intestinal lining.

Holistic remedy - A combined ear, hand and foot reflexology therapy is excellent for relief from constipation. Some clients have found results in one session yet more often it will take several sessions, averaging 4-6 with a professional Reflexologist before a regular elimination routine is established. A monthly reflexology program is suggested once constipation is eliminated to maintain positive results.

Client Observation – Theresa, age 15, has been coming for monthly reflexology session for chronic constipation since 2011. Theresa has seen several gastrointestinal specialists beginning at the age of 8 and after seven years, Theresa still sees her doctor twice a year for monitoring. Theresa takes two types of medications daily to keep her gastrointestinal tract functioning properly. The medications only work 70% of the time for her on days when she is stressed from being overscheduled with school activities and studying, Theresa has found that reflexology has not only helped her find relief, it also helps her relax.

Support Your Liver, Kidney and Spleen Functions

Disorders of the digestive system are extremely common, ranging from the occasional upset stomach to the more life-threatening colorectal cancer. They encompass the gastrointestinal tract as well as the liver, gallbladder, kidney, spleen and pancreas. If you are experiencing poor appetite, this is not a disorder in itself, but usually a symptom of some other problem. It may be related to a digestive system disorder or emotional factors such as depression, illness, stress or trauma.

Liver - The liver helps to digest and metabolize the food we eat, making it the most important organ in the body. If the liver fails, the body begins to fail, too.

Kidney - The kidneys maintain the body's balance (homeostasis), remove waste products, filter the blood, and balance the volume of fluids in the body.

Spleen - The spleen digests food and retrieves nutrients from that food to help your body maintain its strength and health.

Remedy Options

Liver – Eat natural and organic foods rich in antioxidants that will fight disease and toxins. Eating vegetables high in Vitamin B12 also helps the liver in digesting and metabolizing food. Avoid processed foods as well as those with high fat content, and limit alcohol intake.

Kidney – The best foods for the kidney are organic fruits and vegetables, whole grains and low fat dairy. Limit sodium and alcohol intake. Quit smoking and be more physically active.

Spleen - The best foods for the spleen are plain fruits and vegetables, proteins with healthy Omega 3 fatty acids, and plenty of water, anywhere from 8 cups for women and 13 cups for men a day, depending on your level of activities. Avoid fatty food, tobacco and limit alcohol intake.

Holistic remedy - A combined Energy Medicine and ear, hand and foot reflexology therapy has helped many of my clients to encourage toxins to move through digestive tract and filtering organs. With every client, regardless of health or illness, reflexes for filtering organs and gastrointestinal tract are worked on. It takes an average of 4-6 reflexology sessions before filtering organs are supported. Once improvements are routinely apparent, continued monthly maintenance reflexology sessions are recommended to balance filtering organ functions.

Reflexology, Energy Medicine and the Digestive System

What is Reflexology?

Reflexology is a science and an art. It is an ancient healing modality that has been around for more than 5,000 years. It originated in China and Egypt. Reflex points on the feet, hands, and ears represent the body in miniature. The nerve pathways in each foot create an electro-chemical flow that communicates with the entire nervous system. The principal of reflexology is that reflex points and areas, meridian pathways, and chakra (energy centers) regions connect with a specific organ, gland or body part. Through the application of pressure using specific thumb and finger techniques, reflexology works with the peripheral nervous system and encourages the body to relax. Reflexology promotes the reduction of stress, reinforcing the body's ability to stay healthy and vital. This preventative modality encourages wellness through empowerment, understanding how your body can heal, and enabling your body to relax and gain homeostasis.

Reflexology and the Digestive System

Working the reflexology intestinal reflexes in the direction of peristalsis can help move contents through the gastrointestinal tract. The relaxation induced by reflexology helps the body switch over to the parasympathetic nervous system, which supports the whole digestive process. The parasympathetic nervous system is responsible for the unconscious regulation of internal organs and glands. (Breathing, for example, is a parasympathetic process. You would breathe regardless of whether you are conscious about breathing or not.)

- Reflexology promotes the harmonious contraction and relaxation of the diaphragm resulting in a rhythmical massage of the abdominal organs.
- Reflexology helps to release muscular and emotional tension, both of which can severely hamper the digestive process.
- Reflexology can unblock congested energy, promoting a free flow of energy through all channels so that the digestive process from the mouth to the anus can work effectively.
- Reflexology can break down deposits in the feet.
- The stimulation of reflexology decongests energy pathways allowing the digestive system to work optimally (as reflexology does for all bodily systems).

Benefits of Regular Reflexology Sessions

Reduced stress - When the body is stressed, our body's immune system is overworked and overtaxed causing the body to break down. Stimulating reflex points on feet, hands, or ears gives the body the ability to release stress instead of storing it in the organs.

Built-up immune system - When the body is relaxed, the ability to fight off infections increases.

Toxin elimination – One of the biggest killers of the body is the inability to remove toxins efficiently. We are exposed to air, food, electronic, and environmental toxins that the body is removing constantly. By stimulating the reflex points for all the filtering organs, such as the liver, kidney, spleen and lymphatic system, the body's ability to remove toxins is supported.

Improvement in circulation and energy – If waste products and toxins can efficiently be eliminated, your body will have the ability to increase oxygen, blood circulation and your energy level.

Reflexology Tips to Relieve Stomach and Constipation Discomfort

In an average professional reflexology session, approximately fifty-five steps are carried out per foot. Not only are reflex points that address the gastrointestinal system addressed in a 60 minute session but also points impacting the brain and endocrine, reproductive, respiratory, cardiovascular, and musculoskeletal systems. Below are four reflexology steps out of the fifty-five that address stomach, liver, spleen and bowel elimination functions, for you to try at home.

Reflexology 'try-it-yourself' tips

(For a two minute video demonstration on these techniques, visit http://www.youtube.com/watch?v=Zabu4uGqG7c). Looking at the diagrams below, start each of the four sequences with the right foot. Have your left hand support the right foot while the left hand thumb 'walks' with medium pressure along the appropriate location of the foot. After three repeats, switch to the left foot supporting the foot with your right hand, and use your right hand thumb. Perform these four steps once every other day for a week. It will take about three minutes to do these four steps on both feet (1.5 minute per foot). Remember this is only four steps out of fifty-five professional reflexology steps. After your mini self-session, drink plenty of water to encourage intestinal waste to move. If desired results are not achieved, or if more results are desired, call the Healing Place at 508 359-6463 to schedule a professional reflexology session or a 60-minute free consultation.

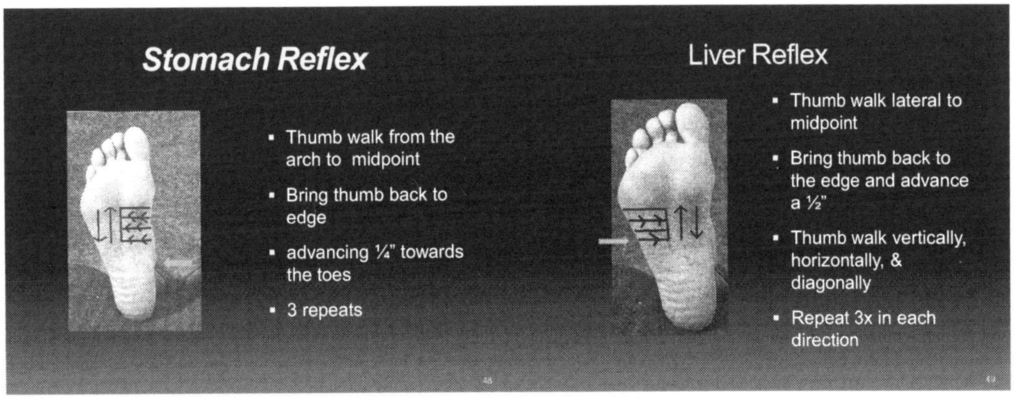

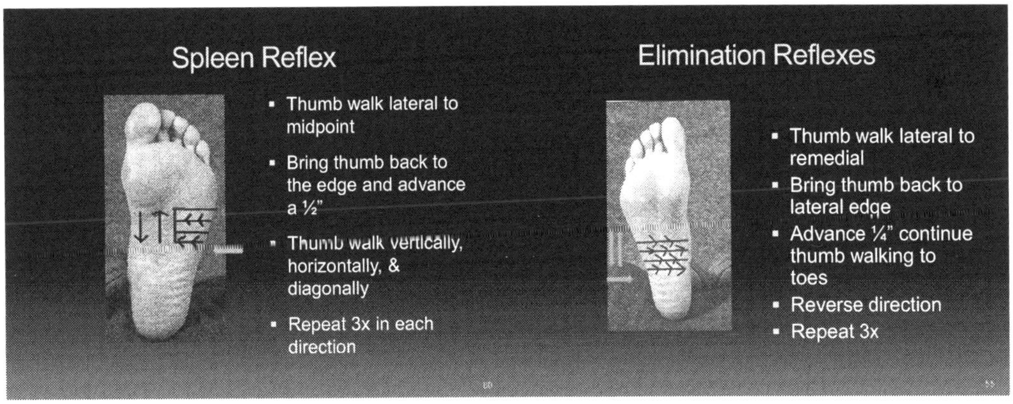

What causes constipation?

- Unbalanced diet - documented by research to be the most important factor in chronic constipation. Foods low in fiber and high fat, such as cheese, meats, and eggs, can cause constipation. Even though you have a craving for bread, spaghetti, and/or sweet foods, it is suggested to try to keep away from processed or white foods and eat whole grains.
- Lack of fiber – people with diets that include a good quantity of fiber are significantly less likely to suffer from constipation. It is suggested that women have 25 grams of fiber a day and men have 38 grams or 14 grams per every 1,000 calories consumed.
- Lack of exercise – poor muscle tone and/or slow or minimal peristalsis (movement of contents through the gastrointestinal tract) increases the likelihood of constipation.
- Miscellaneous other causes - obesity, stress, nerve dysfunction, and habitual use of laxatives.

What is Energy Medicine?

In Energy Medicine, we bring things into "balance" so the body can function more effectively, and simply perform the functions it is meant to, so our bodily systems work together.

When we talk about energy, we are really referring to two kinds of energy fields:

- Putative energy fields – these cannot be measured with traditional technology. These sound energy therapies are created to resonate with the body to promote healing. For example music therapy has shown to lower blood pressure and to reduce pain and anxiety. Treatments include audio techniques such as magnetic, music, radiation, tuning fork therapies.
- Veritable energy fields – these can be measured and include vibration and electromagnetic methods such as visible light and lasers.

Energy Medicine refers to techniques that involve the putative energy fields. Healing methods can use all of the senses - sight, touch, audio, taste and smell. At this time there are no conventional methods to measure this type of energy work other than feedback of clients. By understanding the root of our health issues, we learn where the energy in our body is deficient or excessive. Being conscious of the activities in our lives, we can avoid and remove energy blocks from our bodies and encourage our own healing. Energy healers can normally sense where energies are blocked in the body causing illnesses and health issues.

All living bodies are infused with a "subtle" energy or life force. Energy healers work with the seven main energy centers located on the spine known as "chakras." If our chakras are balanced and open, they help promote general health and wellbeing by ensuring the free flow of life energy throughout the body. When a chakra becomes blocked, damaged, or muddied with residual energy, then our physical and emotional health can be affected. It is believed that blockages in the flow of vital energy eventually result in mental, emotional, and/or physical illness. By removing these blockages and maximizing energy flow we enable the body, mind, and spirit to function optimally.

I have found that most clients' digestive disorders are hereditary. I have also notice that many of these clients have common energy and lifestyle traits. They usually:

- eat on the run
- live stressful lives
- do not have a regular exercise routine
- over-schedule their time
- worry a lot

With digestive disorder cases, energy imbalances show up in the organs in the mid and lower parts of the body which can lead to health issues. Over time, if unprocessed, feelings build up and turn into anger, bitterness and resentment; these emotions can be the seeds to many health issues. I have listed the organs and glands and which emotions impact each one.

Organ or gland	Personality trait	Associated Health Issues
Large Intestine	people who hold on to their past makinginfections, parasites, IBS and colitis and cannot process their "stuff"	them unable to move on
Small Intestine	people who are over stimulated and cannot process their "stuff"	obstructions and diarrhea
Bladder	people with fear of letting go and anxiety	cystitis, infections, stones, and incontinence
Spleen	people with obsessions, harboring old or stagnant thoughts or feelings	autoimmune disorders
Liver	people holding onto anger, or who feel like a victim or feel powerless	hepatitis, cirrhosis, jaundice
Gallbladder	people restraining from expressing rage or bitterness	gallstones
Kidneys	people who hold onto old emotions shame and criticism	kidney stones and renal failure
Stomach	people who have difficulty processing ideas	ulcers and heartburn

People with digestive disorders have a special energy profile about them.

They have a tendency to:

- Overextend themselves to others.
- Be people pleasers.
- Be very empathic, taking on other people's worries and pain.
- Worry about what people think of them.
- Look for self-approval from others.
- Have poor personal boundaries.
- Have one major worry focus (i.e., finance, work, family, mate, etc.).

Benefits of Energy Medicine

Energy Medicine is based upon the principles that the health of the mind, body and spirit is anchored in the body's systems. Since most of us live a very stressful life, it is believed most diseases are stress related and that energy-based therapies can help decrease stress, anxiety and depression.[3]

Energy Medicine lowers blood pressure and slows down breathing. It can also help to turn off the "fight or flight" response caused by stress. It can open energy channels to prevent illnesses. It opens pain centers so that energy flows freely throughout the body and Energy Medicine can boost the immune system by reducing stress.

***Client observation** –Cheryl age 47, has been coming for reflexology since 2006. She suffers from constipation and lower back problems whenever she worries about her finances. Through active energy medicine healing session, Cheryl understood why and where she stores her worries. We were able release her energy blocks through energy medicine after six sessions. Cheryl has been pain free since 2007.*

Conclusion

I hope this information has been helpful in providing insight about what impacts your digestive function--both positively and negatively, and what actions you can take to be in charge of your own healing.

Please remember that this report is strictly informational and not intended for medical purposes or diagnosis; please discuss this information with your health provider before you start any new health regimen.

Need More Help?

This report is only a starting point to give you basic information and tips that you can try. Most people find at least some temporary relief by applying these changes and/or trying reflexology on their own. For quicker and more lasting results, however, consider working with a professional Reflexologist. A certified Reflexologist will not only strengthen your gastrointestinal and elimination reflexes but he/she will perform a complete reflexology protocol that will support your endocrine, respiratory, reproductive, musculoskeletal, cardio, and spinal functions. Before you know it you will feel better, experience more balance and calm, have more normal digestive functioning, and enjoy better sleep.

Looking for *Qualified Care from an Expert*? Call Now For Your Free 60-Minute Consultation!

You don't have to suffer any longer or go it alone in a world of confusing, and sometimes ineffective, medical treatments. Now that you have decided to become proactive with your health care, I can help! I work with clients in my office in Medfield, MA or virtually (via Skype). I would be happy to talk to you about your health issues with a free 60-minute consultation to find out how I can be of service to you, or whether you need other resources that I can recommend. Please call the Healing Place at (508)359-6463.

About the Author

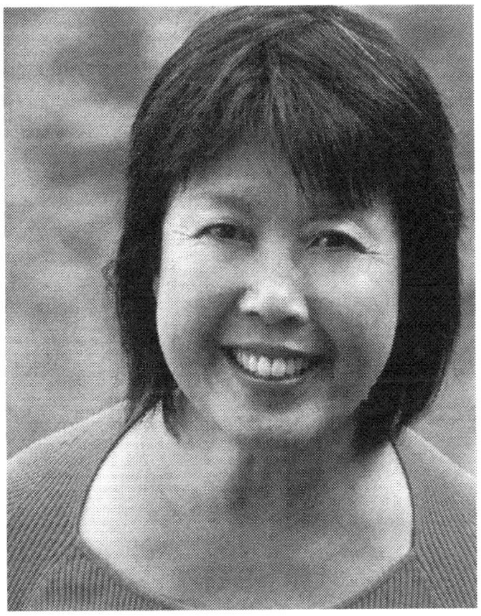

Helen Chin Lui

Helen Chin Lui is highly trained in the field of reflexology with certificates in foot, hand, ear, pediatric, weight management, fertility, musculoskeletal, and canine reflexology from the New England Institute of Reflexology in Wareham, MA. She also earned a certificate to teach an Introduction Relaxation Reflexology program. In 2009, Helen received her certification in Energy Medicine through the 3-year, Rhys Thomas Institute of Energy Medicine in Medway, MA. She also received her Reiki Master certificate from Clear Self Care in Milford, MA.

In addition to offering healing services, where many people have found relief from their physical struggles, including but not limited to pain and embarrassment, Helen teaches energy healing classes at her office in Medfield and at Tri Valley Regional High School in Franklin, MA. She also hosts an educational cable TV show, Holistic Healing, where she talks to experts in various energy healing modalities about their work.

Ms. Lui is in the process of developing a line of self-help-reflexology DVDs to show individuals how to do reflexology themselves at home.

Helen is a member of the Massachusetts Reflexology Association and Reflexology Association of America, as well as an active member of the Dream Factory Community, a woman's support and networking group in Medway, Massachusetts.

References

(1) National Digestive Diseases Information Clearinghouse (NDDIC) 2004 statistics

(2) http://en.wikipedia.org/wiki/Dyspepsia

(3) What is Healing Touch?, Kaiser Permanente, Healthwise Staff, June 29, 2011

Made in the USA
Monee, IL
23 February 2023

28543471R00018